HOME WORKOUT FOR SENIORS OVER 60

Technique to healthy life for seniors

By

JUDITH WALTER

TABLE OF CONTENTS

CHAPTER THREE

- Flexibility and Balance Exercises
- The importance of flexibility and balance exercises for seniors
- Safe and effective exercises for improving flexibility and balance
- Tips for avoiding falls and improving balance at home

CHAPTER FOUR

- Cooling Down and Stretching
- The importance of cooling down and stretching after exercise
- Examples of effective cool-down exercises for seniors
- Safe and effective stretching exercises for seniors over 60

CHAPTER FIVE

- Creating a Home Workout Routine
- Tips for creating a safe and effective home workout routine for seniors over 60
- How to stay motivated and track progress

- Modifications for different fitness levels and health conditions

CONCLUSION

INTRODUCTION

As we age, it becomes increasingly important to maintain an active lifestyle to maintain our physical and mental well-being. Regular exercise is one of the most effective ways to stay healthy as we get older. In this book,we will discuss the benefits of regular exercise for seniors.

Maintains Muscle Mass and Strength
As we age, our muscle mass and strength tend to decline, leading to reduced mobility and increased risk of falls. Regular exercise, particularly strength training, can help prevent these negative outcomes by maintaining and even increasing muscle mass and strength. This, in turn, can improve overall mobility and reduce the risk of falls.

Improves Cardiovascular Health
Regular exercise can help improve cardiovascular health, reducing the risk of heart disease, stroke, and other cardiovascular

conditions. Exercise helps to strengthen the heart and blood vessels, improving blood flow and oxygen delivery to the body's tissues.

Helps Control Chronic Conditions
Exercise has been shown to help control chronic conditions such as diabetes, arthritis, and osteoporosis. For example, regular exercise can help improve insulin sensitivity and blood sugar control in those with diabetes. It can also help maintain bone density and reduce the risk of fractures in those with osteoporosis.

Reduces Risk of Cognitive Decline
Studies have shown that regular exercise can help reduce the risk of cognitive decline and dementia in older adults. Exercise may help improve cognitive function by increasing blood flow and oxygen delivery to the brain, as well as promoting the growth of new brain cells.

Improves Mood and Reduces Stress
Regular exercise can also improve mood and reduce stress in older adults. Exercise has been

shown to increase the production of endorphins, which are natural mood boosters. It can also help reduce levels of stress hormones such as cortisol.

Finally, regular exercise can provide social benefits for seniors. Participating in group exercise classes or activities can help seniors meet new people and form friendships, reducing feelings of social isolation and loneliness.

In conclusion, regular exercise is essential for seniors to maintain their physical and mental health. It can help maintain muscle mass and strength, improve cardiovascular health, control chronic conditions, reduce the risk of cognitive decline, improve mood, and provide social benefits. It's never too late to start exercising, and even small amounts of physical activity can make a big difference in overall health and well-being.

CORE STRENGTH AND AGING.

As we age, our bodies undergo a series of natural changes that can significantly impact our physical function and quality of life. One of the most crucial aspects of maintaining good health and independence in our senior years is maintaining core strength. The core muscles, including those in the abdomen, back, hips, and pelvis, play a crucial role in maintaining balance, stability, and movement control. However, as we age, these muscles naturally weaken, leading to a range of physical limitations and health concerns.

In this book, we will explore the aging process and its impact on core strength in seniors over the age of 60. We will delve into the science behind muscle loss and changes in bone density and joint mobility, as well as the effects of a sedentary lifestyle and poor nutrition on core strength. We will also provide practical strategies for improving and maintaining core strength, including strength training exercises, yoga, and Pilates, as well as tips for healthy eating and lifestyle habits.

Whether you are a senior looking to maintain your independence and quality of life, a caregiver seeking to support the health and well-being of a loved one, or a healthcare professional working with older adults, this book will provide valuable insights and strategies for improving core strength and overall physical function in seniors over 60.

CORE MUSCLES AND HEALTH

The core muscles play a critical role in maintaining overall health and wellness. These muscles, which include the muscles of the abdomen, back, hips, and pelvis, provide support and stability for the spine and pelvis, help maintain good posture, and facilitate proper movement patterns.

Strong core muscles can also reduce the risk of injury, particularly in the lower back and hips. By providing support and stability to these areas, strong core muscles can help prevent falls, strains, and other injuries.

Additionally, research has shown that maintaining good core strength can improve athletic performance, particularly in sports that require quick, explosive movements or changes in direction. Strong core muscles can also help improve balance and coordination, making it easier to perform daily activities and reduce the risk of falls.

In addition to physical health benefits, good core strength can also have a positive impact on mental health. Good posture and strong core muscles can boost confidence and self-esteem, while reducing pain and discomfort in the lower back and hips can improve overall quality of life.

Overall, maintaining good core strength is essential for maintaining good health and wellness. Incorporating exercises that target the core muscles into your regular fitness routine, such as planks, crunches, and squats, can help improve core strength and reduce the risk of injury and discomfort.

CHAPTER ONE

THE AGING PROCESS AND ITS IMPACT
The aging process is a natural and inevitable part of life that affects everyone, and it can have a significant impact on core strength in seniors over the age of 60. As people age, their muscles, including those in the core, tend to weaken and lose mass, which can result in a decreased ability to perform daily tasks and engage in physical activity.

One of the main reasons for this decline in core strength is sarcopenia, which is the age-related loss of muscle mass and strength. Sarcopenia can begin as early as age 30 and can accelerate after age 60. This loss of muscle mass can lead to a decrease in core strength, as the core muscles play an essential role in maintaining stability and balance.

Another factor that can contribute to a decline in core strength in seniors is a sedentary lifestyle. Many older adults may become less active as they age, which can lead to muscle loss and a decline in core strength. A lack of physical activity can also increase the risk of falls and injuries, which can further impact core strength.

Fortunately, there are steps that seniors can take to maintain or improve their core strength as they age. Regular exercise that includes strength training and core-focused exercises can help to build and maintain muscle mass and improve core strength. Activities such as yoga, Pilates, and Tai Chi can be particularly beneficial for seniors, as they focus on building core strength and improving balance and flexibility.

In addition to exercise, a healthy diet that includes plenty of protein can also help to maintain muscle mass and improve core strength. Seniors should aim to consume a balanced diet that includes lean protein sources such as fish, chicken, and beans, as well as plenty of fruits and vegetables.

Overall, while aging can impact core strength in seniors over the age of 60, there are steps that can be taken to maintain or improve core strength and overall health. Regular exercise and a healthy diet can help to prevent muscle loss and improve balance and stability, enabling older adults to maintain their independence and enjoy an active lifestyle.

THE SCIENCE BEHIND MUSCLE LOSS AND CHANGES IN BONE DENSITY AND JOINT MOBILITY

Muscle loss, changes in bone density, and joint mobility are all natural aspects of the aging process, and they are influenced by a variety of physiological and lifestyle factors.

Muscle loss, or sarcopenia, occurs as people age, and it is primarily caused by a decline in the production of anabolic hormones such as testosterone, insulin-like growth factor 1 (IGF-1), and growth hormone. This decline in hormone production leads to a reduction in muscle mass, strength, and power. Additionally, inactivity and poor nutrition can accelerate the loss of muscle mass and function.

Changes in bone density, or osteoporosis, is another common age-related issue. As people age, their bones become less dense and more fragile, increasing the risk of fractures and falls. This loss of bone density is influenced by several factors, including hormonal changes, such as decreased estrogen production in women, and a decrease in calcium absorption by the body. Additionally, inactivity and poor nutrition can also contribute to the loss of bone density.

Joint mobility can also decline as people age. This can be caused by a variety of factors, including wear and tear on the joints, loss of cartilage, inflammation, and reduced flexibility due to reduced muscle mass and strength. Arthritis is also a common condition that affects joint mobility in older adults.

Fortunately, there are ways to mitigate the negative effects of aging on muscle mass, bone density, and joint mobility. Regular exercise, particularly strength training and weight-bearing exercises, can help to preserve muscle mass and improve bone density. A healthy diet that includes adequate protein, calcium, and vitamin D is also important for maintaining muscle and bone health. Additionally, maintaining an active lifestyle can help to prevent joint stiffness and maintain joint mobility.

In summary, muscle loss, changes in bone density, and joint mobility are all natural aspects of the aging process that can be influenced by a variety of factors. However, regular exercise and a healthy lifestyle can help to mitigate these effects and improve overall health and quality of life in older adults.

THE EFFECTS OF A SEDENTARY LIFESTYLE AND POOR NUTRITION ON CORE STRENGTH.

A sedentary lifestyle and poor nutrition can have significant negative effects on core strength, which can impact an individual's ability to perform daily activities and engage in physical activity.

When someone leads a sedentary lifestyle, it means they are not engaging in enough physical activity throughout the day. This lack of movement and exercise can result in a loss of muscle mass and strength, including the core muscles. The core muscles are essential for maintaining posture, balance, and stability, and a lack of strength in these muscles can lead to a higher risk of falls, back pain, and other issues.

Poor nutrition can also negatively impact core strength. A diet that is low in protein and essential nutrients can lead to muscle loss, weakness, and atrophy, which can affect core strength. Additionally, a diet high in sugar and unhealthy fats can lead to weight gain, which can put additional stress on the core muscles and lead to further weakness and loss of strength.

Together, a sedentary lifestyle and poor nutrition can create a cycle of muscle loss, weakness, and poor health outcomes. Individuals who are not engaging in enough physical activity and consuming a balanced diet may experience a reduction in core strength and overall muscle mass, which can lead to a reduced ability to perform daily tasks and engage in physical activity. This can lead to a further decline in health, as well as a higher risk of chronic diseases such as heart disease, diabetes, and obesity.

Fortunately, there are steps that individuals can take to improve their core strength, even if they have been leading a sedentary lifestyle and consuming a poor diet. Engaging in regular exercise that focuses on core strength, such as Pilates or yoga, can help to improve muscle mass and strength in the core muscles. Additionally, consuming a balanced diet that includes lean protein sources, healthy fats, and essential nutrients can provide the body with the fuel it needs to build and maintain muscle mass and strength. By making lifestyle changes and prioritizing physical activity and nutrition, individuals can improve their core strength and overall health outcomes.

PRACTICAL STRATEGIES FOR IMPROVING AND MAINTAINING CORE

Improving and maintaining core strength is important for overall health and can help prevent injuries and chronic pain. Here are some practical strategies for improving and maintaining core strength:

✓ Engage in targeted exercises: There are many exercises that specifically target the core muscles, such as planks, sit-ups, and leg lifts. Incorporating these exercises into a workout routine can help to improve core strength over time. It's important to start with basic exercises and gradually increase difficulty to avoid injury.

✓ Use stability balls: Stability balls can be used to perform a variety of exercises that target the core muscles. Using a stability ball for exercises such as crunches or push-ups can increase the intensity of the workout and improve core strength.

✓ Practice yoga or Pilates: Both yoga and Pilates focus on building core strength and stability through a variety of exercises and movements. These practices can improve balance, posture, and overall body awareness, which can lead to improved core strength.

✓ Incorporate resistance training: Resistance training, such as weightlifting or resistance band exercises, can improve overall muscle mass and strength, including the core muscles. Adding resistance training to a workout routine can help to build and maintain core strength over time.

✓ Focus on posture: Maintaining good posture throughout the day can help to strengthen the core muscles and prevent back pain. Practicing good posture during activities such as sitting, standing, and walking can help to engage the core muscles and improve overall core strength.

✓ Pay attention to nutrition: Consuming a balanced diet that includes lean protein sources, healthy fats, and essential nutrients can provide the body with the fuel it needs to build and maintain muscle mass and strength, including the core muscles.

✓ Stay active: Engaging in regular physical activity, such as walking, cycling, or swimming, can help to maintain overall muscle mass and strength, including the core muscles. Incorporating physical activity into daily routines can improve overall health outcomes and maintain core strength over time.

Incorporating these strategies into a regular routine can help to improve and maintain core strength and overall health outcomes. Remember to start slow and gradually increase difficulty to avoid injury, and always consult with a healthcare professional before starting a new exercise routine.

CHAPTER TWO

WORKOUT STREACHING WARM UP ROUTINE

A good workout stretching warm-up routine is essential for preventing injuries, preparing your body for physical activity, and improving your overall performance during exercise. A proper warm-up routine typically involves a series of exercises that gradually increase your heart rate and breathing, mobilize your joints, and stretch your muscles.

A basic warm-up routine might include a few minutes of light cardio exercise, such as jogging in place or jumping jacks, to get your heart rate up and your blood flowing. This can be followed by some dynamic stretching exercises, such as leg swings, arm circles, or hip rotations, to mobilize your joints and increase flexibility.

Once you've completed the initial warm-up exercises, you can move on to some targeted stretching exercises to prepare your muscles for the upcoming workout. Some examples of good stretches include:

✓ Hamstring stretch: Stand with your feet shoulder-width apart and stretch your arms towards the ceiling. Slowly bend forward from the hips and reach towards your toes, keeping your knees slightly bent.

✓ Quadriceps stretch: Stand with your feet hip-width apart and hold onto a stable surface for balance. Bend your right knee and bring your heel towards your buttocks, then grasp your ankle with your right hand and hold for 10-15 seconds. Repeat on the other side.

✓ Shoulder stretch: Stand with your feet shoulder-width apart and interlace your fingers behind your back. Slowly lift your arms towards the ceiling and hold for 10-15 seconds.

✓ Calf stretch: Stand with your feet shoulder-width apart and step your right foot forward. Keep your left leg straight and your left heel on the ground, then lean forward towards your right knee. Hold for 10-15 seconds, then repeat on the other side.

✓ Chest stretch: Stand with your feet shoulder-width apart and interlace your fingers behind your back. Slowly lift your arms towards the ceiling and squeeze your shoulder blades together. Hold for 10-15 seconds.

Remember to breathe deeply and focus on relaxing your muscles as you perform these stretches. Taking the time to properly warm up and stretch before your workout can help prevent injury, improve your performance, and make your workout more enjoyable overall.

WARM-UP EXERCISES.
Jumping jacks - Start with your feet together and arms by your sides. Jump and spread your feet while raising your arms overhead. Then jump back to the starting position.

Lunges - Take a big step forward with one foot and lower your body until your front knee is bent at a 90-degree angle. Keep your back straight and your front knee over your ankle.

Arm circles - Stand with your feet shoulder-width apart and raise your arms straight out to your sides. Make small circles with your arms, gradually increasing the size of the circles.

High knees - Stand with your feet hip-width apart and lift your knees up towards your chest, alternating between each leg.

Squats - Stand with your feet shoulder-width apart and lower your body as if you were sitting back in a chair. Keep your back straight and your knees over your ankles.

Remember to start slowly and gradually increase the intensity and duration of your warm-up exercises. It's important to warm up before any physical activity to prevent injury and improve performance.

WHY WARM-UP EXERCISES

Warm-up exercises are important for seniors for several reasons:

Improved circulation: As we age, our circulation slows down, and warming up can help improve blood flow to our muscles, making them more flexible and less prone to injury.

Injury prevention: Warm-up exercises can help seniors avoid muscle strains and other injuries by preparing their bodies for physical activity. A proper warm-up helps to loosen the muscles, increase flexibility and reduce stiffness.

Improved balance: Older adults are at a higher risk of falls due to loss of balance. A warm-up that includes balance exercises can help improve coordination and stability, reducing the risk of falls.

Improved joint mobility: As we age, our joints become stiffer and less flexible. Warm-up exercises can help improve joint mobility, reducing the risk of arthritis and other joint-related problems.

Improved mental focus: Engaging in a warm-up routine before any physical activity can help seniors feel more alert and focused. This can be particularly important for seniors who may have difficulty concentrating due to age-related changes in cognitive function.

Overall, warm-up exercises are an important part of any senior's fitness routine. They can help improve overall health, reduce the risk of injury, and make physical activity more enjoyable.

THE EFFECTIVE WARM-UP EXERCISES FOR SENIORS OVER 60

As we age, it becomes increasingly important to take care of our bodies, and warming up before physical activity is essential for seniors over 60. A proper warm-up routine can help improve circulation, prevent injury, improve balance and joint mobility, and enhance mental focus. Here

are some effective warm-up exercises for seniors
over 60:

Walking: Walking is a low-impact exercise that
is easy on the joints and provides an excellent
warm-up for seniors. Start by walking at a slow
pace for a few minutes and gradually increase
the pace as you feel more comfortable.

Arm circles: Stand with your feet shoulder-width
apart and raise your arms straight out to your
sides. Make small circles with your arms,
gradually increasing the size of the circles. This
exercise helps to loosen up the shoulder joints
and improve mobility.

Leg swings: Stand facing a wall or a sturdy
object and gently swing one leg forward and
backward, then side to side. This exercise helps
to warm up the hip joints and improve balance.

Chair squats: Stand in front of a chair and slowly
lower your body as if you were sitting back in
the chair. Keep your back straight and your

knees over your ankles. This exercise helps to warm up the lower body and improve leg strength.

Calf raises: Stand with your feet shoulder-width apart and slowly rise up onto the balls of your feet, then lower back down. This exercise helps to warm up the calves and improve balance.

Shoulder rolls: Stand with your feet shoulder-width apart and roll your shoulders forward and backward in a circular motion. This exercise helps to warm up the shoulder joints and improve mobility.

Toe taps: Stand with your feet shoulder-width apart and tap your toes alternately on the ground. This exercise helps to warm up the ankles and improve balance.

Remember to start slowly and gradually increase the intensity and duration of your warm-up exercises. It's important to listen to your body and stop if you feel any discomfort or pain. A proper warm-up routine can help seniors over 60 stay active, healthy, and independent.

THE IMPORTANCE OF FINDING SAFE AND EFFECTIVE HOME WORKOUT ROUTINES

In recent years, home workout routines have become increasingly popular as people seek convenient and cost-effective ways to stay active and healthy. However, with the rise of home workouts comes the need to find safe and effective routines that can be done at home without risking injury or wasting time on ineffective exercises. In this book, we will discuss the importance of finding safe and effective home workout routines.

PREVENTING INJURY

One of the most important reasons to find safe and effective home workout routines is to prevent injury. Without proper guidance and instruction, it's easy to perform exercises incorrectly and put unnecessary strain on the body, leading to injury. By finding safe and effective routines that are appropriate for your fitness level and goals, you can minimize the risk of injury and ensure that you're exercising safely.

MAXIMIZING RESULTS

Another reason to find safe and effective home workout routines is to maximize the results of your workouts. If you're spending time and effort on exercises that aren't effective or don't challenge your body, you're not going to see the results you're hoping for. By finding routines that are designed to challenge your body and help you achieve your fitness goals, you can ensure that you're making the most of your workouts.

SAVING TIME

Home workouts can be a great way to save time and avoid the hassle of going to a gym or fitness class. However, if you're not following a safe and effective routine, you may end up wasting time on exercises that aren't getting you closer to your goals. By finding routines that are designed

to be efficient and effective, you can save time
and get a great workout in the comfort of your
own home.

STAYING MOTIVATED

Finally, finding safe and effective home workout
routines can help you stay motivated and
committed to your fitness goals. When you're
seeing results and feeling challenged by your
workouts, it's easier to stay motivated and stick
to your routine. On the other hand, if you're not
seeing results or feeling bored with your
workouts, you may be more likely to give up or
skip workouts altogether.

In conclusion, finding safe and effective home
workout routines is crucial for anyone looking to
stay active and healthy at home. By prioritizing
safety, effectiveness, efficiency, and motivation,
you can find routines that are tailored to your
goals and fitness level, helping you achieve the
results you're looking for while minimizing the
risk of injury. With the right home workout
routine, you can stay active and healthy while

enjoying the convenience and comfort of working out at home.

STRENGTH TRAINING FOR SENIORS

Strength training is an essential part of maintaining physical health and well-being, especially for seniors over the age of 60. As we age, our bodies experience a natural decline in muscle mass and bone density, which can increase the risk of falls and fractures. However, incorporating strength training into our fitness routine can help to build and maintain muscle mass, improve balance, and reduce the risk of injury. In this way, strength training can provide numerous benefits for seniors, including increased mobility, independence, and overall quality of life. Whether you're a seasoned athlete or new to exercise, strength training is an excellent way to support your long-term health and wellness.

THE IMPORTANCE OF STRENGTH TRAINING FOR SENIORS

Strength training is crucial for seniors because it can help them maintain their physical health and independence as they age. Here are some key reasons why strength training is essential for seniors:

Builds muscle mass: As we age, we naturally lose muscle mass, which can lead to weakness and an increased risk of falls. Strength training helps to build and maintain muscle mass, which can improve overall strength and balance.

Improves bone density: Bone density decreases with age, which can lead to osteoporosis and an increased risk of fractures. Strength training can help improve bone density and reduce the risk of osteoporosis.

Increases metabolism: Strength training can help increase metabolism, which can aid in weight management and reduce the risk of obesity-related health problems.

Enhances mobility: Strength training can improve overall mobility, making it easier to perform daily tasks such as climbing stairs or carrying groceries.

Reduces risk of injury: Strength training can help improve balance and coordination, reducing the risk of falls and injuries.

Improves overall quality of life: Regular strength training can help seniors feel stronger, more energetic, and more independent, improving overall quality of life.

In conclusion, strength training is incredibly important for seniors, and can help maintain their physical health and independence as they age. By incorporating strength training into their fitness routine, seniors can experience numerous benefits and enjoy a better quality of life.

SAFE AND EFFECTIVE STRENGTH TRAINING EXERCISES FOR SENIORS

When it comes to strength training for seniors over 60, it's essential to prioritize safety and choose exercises that are appropriate for their fitness level and physical abilities. Here are some safe and effective strength training exercises for seniors:

Bodyweight squats: Squats can help strengthen the legs and glutes, which are important for balance and mobility. Seniors can start with bodyweight squats and progress to using a chair for support if necessary.

Seated leg press: The seated leg press is an excellent exercise for seniors as it targets the legs and glutes while providing support for the lower back. This exercise can be performed on a weight machine or with resistance bands.

Wall push-ups: Wall push-ups are a safe and effective exercise for seniors as they target the chest, shoulders, and triceps without putting too much strain on the joints. Seniors can start with a wall push-up and progress to a counter push-up or a regular push-up if they are able.

Bicep curls: Bicep curls can help strengthen the arms and improve grip strength, which is essential for daily activities such as opening jars or carrying groceries. Seniors can use dumbbells or resistance bands to perform bicep curls.

Step-ups: Step-ups are a great exercise for building leg strength and improving balance. Seniors can use a step or a sturdy bench to perform step-ups.

Planks: Planks are a safe and effective exercise for strengthening the core muscles, which are essential for balance and stability. Seniors can start with a modified plank on their knees and progress to a full plank as they get stronger.

It's important for seniors to start with a lower weight or resistance level and gradually increase as they get stronger. It's also essential to prioritize proper form and technique to prevent injury. A certified personal trainer or physical therapist can help seniors develop a safe and effective strength training program.

USING HOUSEHOLD ITEMS AS WEIGHTS FOR STRENGTH TRAINING

Using household items as weights for strength training is an excellent way to stay active and fit, especially for seniors who may not have access to a gym or traditional workout equipment. Here are some household items that can be used as weights for strength training:

Water bottles: Filled water bottles can be used as light weights for exercises such as bicep curls or shoulder presses.

Canned goods: Canned goods such as beans or soup cans can be used as weights for exercises such as tricep extensions or lateral raises.

Towels: A towel can be used for resistance exercises such as towel bicep curls or towel rows.

Backpack: A backpack filled with books or other heavy items can be used as a weight for exercises such as squats or lunges.

Chair: A sturdy chair can be used for exercises such as seated leg extensions or dips.

It's important to note that household items may not be as sturdy or as evenly weighted as traditional weights, so it's important to start with lighter weights and focus on proper form and technique to prevent injury. A certified personal trainer or physical therapist can provide guidance on how to safely and effectively use household items for strength training.

CHAPTER THREE

CARDIO EXERCISE BENEFITS.

Cardiovascular exercise, also known as aerobic exercise, is any type of physical activity that raises your heart rate and breathing rate, and increases oxygen consumption in your body. Examples of cardiovascular exercise include running, cycling, swimming, rowing, dancing, brisk walking, and jumping rope.

Regular cardiovascular exercise has many benefits for your overall health and well-being, including:

Improving cardiovascular health: Regular cardio exercise can improve the health of your heart and blood vessels, reducing your risk of heart disease, stroke, and high blood pressure.

Burning calories: Cardio exercise can help you burn calories and lose weight, which can also help reduce your risk of obesity-related health problems.

Boosting mood: Cardio exercise has been shown to release endorphins, the body's natural "feel-good" chemicals, which can improve mood and reduce feelings of anxiety and depression.

Strengthening bones and muscles: Cardio exercise can help strengthen your bones and muscles, which can improve your balance and reduce your risk of falls and fractures.

Improving sleep: Regular cardio exercise can help improve the quality and duration of your sleep, which can have a positive impact on your overall health and well-being.

It's recommended that adults aim for at least 150 minutes of moderate-intensity cardio exercise or 75 minutes of vigorous-intensity cardio exercise per week, along with muscle-strengthening activities at least two days per week. However, it's important to check with your doctor before starting any new exercise program, especially if you have any underlying health conditions or concerns.

THE BENEFITS OF CARDIOVASCULAR EXERCISE FOR SENIORS

Cardiovascular exercise is particularly beneficial for seniors as it can help improve overall health, mobility, and quality of life. Here are some of the benefits of cardiovascular exercise for seniors:

Improves cardiovascular health: Cardiovascular exercise can help improve heart health by increasing heart rate and blood flow, reducing the risk of heart disease and stroke.

Increases endurance and stamina: Regular cardio exercise can increase endurance and stamina, making it easier to perform everyday activities such as walking, climbing stairs, and carrying groceries.

Reduces the risk of falls: Cardiovascular exercise can help improve balance and stability, reducing the risk of falls and injuries.

Boosts mood and cognitive function: Cardio exercise releases endorphins, which can help improve mood and reduce feelings of anxiety and depression. It can also improve cognitive function, including memory and decision-making.

Improves sleep quality: Regular cardio exercise can help improve sleep quality, which can lead to improved overall health and well-being.

Supports healthy weight management: Cardiovascular exercise can help burn calories and support healthy weight management, which can reduce the risk of obesity-related health problems.

Reduces the risk of chronic diseases: Regular cardio exercise can help reduce the risk of chronic diseases such as diabetes, high blood pressure, and certain types of cancer.

It's important for seniors to speak with their doctor before beginning any new exercise program, and to start gradually and work at a comfortable pace. Activities such as walking, swimming, cycling, and low-impact aerobics are generally safe and effective forms of cardiovascular exercise for seniors.

SAFE AND EFFECTIVE CARDIOVASCULAR EXERCISES FOR SENIORS

There are several safe and effective cardiovascular exercises that seniors over 60 can do to improve their overall health and well-being. It's important to start slowly and work up gradually, and to always consult with a doctor before beginning any new exercise program. Here are some examples of safe and effective cardiovascular exercises for seniors over 60:

Walking: Walking is a low-impact exercise that is easy on the joints and can be done almost anywhere. Seniors can start with short walks and gradually increase the duration and intensity over time.

Swimming: Swimming is a low-impact exercise that is easy on the joints and can help improve cardiovascular health. It's also a great option for seniors with mobility issues.

Cycling: Cycling is a low-impact exercise that can help improve cardiovascular health and leg strength. Seniors can start with a stationary bike and gradually work up to riding outdoors.

Low-impact aerobics: Low-impact aerobics are a great way to improve cardiovascular health and overall fitness. Seniors can find classes specifically designed for their age group.

Dancing: Dancing is a fun way to get cardiovascular exercise and improve balance and coordination. Seniors can take dance classes or dance at home to their favorite music.

Chair exercises: Chair exercises are low-impact exercises that can be done while sitting in a chair. They can help improve cardiovascular health and overall fitness, and are a great option for seniors with mobility issues.

Tai chi: Tai chi is a low-impact exercise that can help improve balance, coordination, and overall fitness. It's also a great option for seniors with mobility issues.

Remember to always warm up before exercising, stay hydrated, and listen to your body. If you experience pain or discomfort, stop exercising and speak with your doctor.

HOW TO INCORPORATE CARDIO INTO A HOME WORKOUT ROUTINE

Incorporating cardio into a home workout routine is easier than you might think. Here are some tips to help you get started:

Choose a cardio exercise: There are many cardio exercises that can be done at home, such as jumping jacks, running in place, jumping rope, or dancing. Choose an exercise that you enjoy and that suits your fitness level.

Schedule your workout: Set aside time in your day to exercise, and make it a priority. Aim for at least 30 minutes of cardio exercise most days of the week.

Warm up: Before starting your cardio workout, warm up your body by doing some gentle stretches or low-intensity exercises for 5-10 minutes.

Use equipment if necessary: If you have equipment such as a stationary bike or a treadmill at home, incorporate it into your workout routine. If you don't have equipment, you can still get a great cardio workout using your own body weight.

Mix it up: To keep things interesting, mix up your cardio exercises. Try different exercises on different days or incorporate intervals of high-intensity exercise followed by periods of low-intensity exercise.

Cool down and stretch: After your cardio workout, cool down with some low-intensity exercise and then do some stretching to help prevent muscle soreness.

Stay motivated: To stay motivated, try working out with a friend or using an app or online program that provides guidance and accountability.

Remember to always listen to your body, start slowly and gradually increase the intensity and duration of your workout over time. Also, make sure to check with your doctor before beginning any new exercise program, especially if you have any underlying health conditions or concerns.

CHAPTER FOUR

FLEXIBILITY AND BALANCE EXERCISES.

Flexibility and balance exercises are important for maintaining overall fitness and reducing the risk of injury. Here are some examples of exercises you can do to improve your flexibility and balance:

Yoga: Yoga is a great way to improve flexibility and balance. There are many different types of yoga, but all of them involve stretching and holding poses that improve flexibility, strength, and balance.

Tai chi: Tai chi is a Chinese martial art that is also a great form of exercise for improving balance and flexibility. Tai chi involves slow, flowing movements that improve balance, coordination, and strength.

Pilates: Pilates is a low-impact exercise that focuses on strengthening the core muscles and improving flexibility and balance. Pilates exercises can be done on a mat or using equipment such as a reformer.

Stretching: Stretching is a simple and effective way to improve flexibility. You can do static stretches (holding a stretch for a period of time) or dynamic stretches (moving through a range of motion) to improve your flexibility.

Balance exercises: There are many different types of balance exercises you can do to improve your balance, such as standing on one leg, heel-to-toe walks, and balance boards. These exercises can help improve your balance and reduce the risk of falls.

Remember to always warm up before doing any exercise and to consult with a doctor or fitness professional before starting a new exercise program.

THE IMPORTANCE OF FLEXIBILITY AND BALANCE EXERCISES FOR SENIORS

Flexibility and balance exercises are particularly important for seniors because as we age, our muscles and joints become less flexible, and our balance can deteriorate. This can increase the risk of falls and injuries, which can be particularly dangerous for seniors. Here are some reasons why flexibility and balance exercises are especially important for seniors:

Reducing the risk of falls: Falls are a common and serious problem for seniors. By improving balance and flexibility, seniors can reduce their risk of falling and improve their ability to recover from a fall if one does occur.

Maintaining independence: Loss of balance and mobility can make it difficult for seniors to perform everyday activities such as walking, climbing stairs, and getting up from a chair. By improving flexibility and balance, seniors can maintain their independence and continue to perform these activities with ease.

Reducing pain and stiffness: As we age, our muscles and joints can become stiff and painful. Stretching exercises can help to reduce this stiffness and improve range of motion, making it easier to move around and perform everyday activities.

Improving posture: Poor posture can contribute to pain and discomfort, especially in the neck, back, and hips. Flexibility exercises can help improve posture and reduce pain in these areas.

Enhancing overall fitness: Flexibility and balance exercises are a great way to stay active and maintain overall fitness. By staying active, seniors can improve their cardiovascular health, maintain a healthy weight, and reduce the risk of chronic diseases such as diabetes and heart disease.

Overall, flexibility and balance exercises are important for seniors to maintain their health, independence, and quality of life. It's important to consult with a doctor or fitness professional before starting a new exercise program to ensure safety and effectiveness.

SAFE AND EFFECTIVE EXERCISES FOR IMPROVING FLEXIBILITY AND BALANCE

There are many safe and effective exercises that can help improve flexibility and balance. Here are some examples:

Leg stretches: Sit on the floor with your legs extended in front of you. Reach forward and try to touch your toes, holding the stretch for 15-30 seconds. You can also try seated butterfly stretches or seated spinal twists.

Hip stretches: Sit on the floor with your legs crossed in front of you. Gently press down on your knees to open up your hips. Hold the stretch for 15-30 seconds. You can also try hip flexor stretches or figure-four stretches.

Standing calf stretches: Stand facing a wall and place your hands on the wall. Step back with one foot, keeping it flat on the ground, and bend your front knee. Hold the stretch for 15-30 seconds and then switch sides.

One-legged balance exercises: Stand on one leg and hold the position for 30 seconds. Repeat on the other leg. You can also try standing on a pillow or a balance board to make the exercise more challenging.

Yoga poses: Yoga is a great way to improve flexibility and balance. Poses such as downward-facing dog, warrior II, and tree pose can help improve balance and flexibility.

Tai chi movements: Tai chi movements involve slow, flowing movements that improve balance, coordination, and strength. You can follow along with a tai chi video or take a tai chi class to learn the movements.

Remember to always warm up before doing any exercise and to consult with a doctor or fitness professional before starting a new exercise program. It's important to start slowly and gradually increase the intensity and duration of your workouts to avoid injury.

TIPS FOR AVOIDING FALLS AND IMPROVING BALANCE AT HOME

Falls are a common and serious problem, especially for seniors. However, there are many things you can do to avoid falls and improve balance at home. Here are some tips:

Remove tripping hazards: Clear your home of any tripping hazards such as loose rugs, clutter, and electrical cords. Make sure all walkways are well-lit and free of obstacles.

Use assistive devices: If you have difficulty walking or maintaining your balance, consider using assistive devices such as canes, walkers, or grab bars in the bathroom.

Wear appropriate footwear: Wear shoes with non-slip soles and good support. Avoid wearing shoes with high heels or slippery soles.

Improve lighting: Make sure all areas of your home are well-lit. Install nightlights in hallways and bathrooms to help you navigate at night.

Exercise regularly: Regular exercise, including flexibility and balance exercises, can help improve your balance and reduce the risk of falls. Consider taking a fitness class or working with a personal trainer to develop an exercise program that is right for you.

Stay hydrated: Dehydration can cause dizziness and affect your balance. Make sure you drink plenty of water throughout the day.

Get regular check-ups: Regular check-ups with your doctor can help identify any health problems that may affect your balance, such as vision or ear problems.

By taking these steps, you can reduce your risk of falls and improve your balance, allowing you to maintain your independence and quality of life.

CHAPTER FIVE

COOLING & STRETCHING

Cooling down and stretching are important parts of any workout routine. Cooling down refers to the gradual reduction of exercise intensity and allowing the body to return to its pre-workout state, while stretching involves elongating the muscles to increase flexibility and range of motion.

HERE ARE SOME BENEFITS OF COOLING DOWN AND STRETCHING:

Reduces risk of injury: Cooling down and stretching can help to reduce the risk of injury by allowing the body to gradually return to its pre-workout state and decreasing the chances of muscles or joints becoming stiff or sore.

Improves flexibility: Stretching helps to increase flexibility and range of motion, which can lead to improved athletic performance and reduced risk of injury.

Aids in recovery: Cooling down and stretching can help to remove waste products such as lactic acid from the muscles, reducing soreness and aiding in recovery.

Reduces stress: Cooling down and stretching can help to reduce stress levels, promoting relaxation and a sense of well-being.

Some examples of cooling down and stretching exercises include:

Walking or jogging at a slower pace for 5-10 minutes
Gentle yoga poses, such as downward dog or child's pose
Static stretching exercises, such as hamstring stretches or quad stretches, held for 20-30 seconds
Foam rolling, using a foam roller to massage and release tight muscles.
Remember to always listen to your body and stretch within your limits. It's also important to

speak with your healthcare provider before starting any new exercise routine.

THE IMPORTANCE OF COOLING DOWN AND STRETCHING AFTER EXERCISE

Cooling down and stretching after exercise are important because they help your body transition from a state of exertion to a state of rest. Here are some of the main benefits of cooling down and stretching after exercise:

Helps prevent injury: After a workout, your muscles are warm and more pliable, making them more susceptible to injury. By cooling down and stretching, you can help prevent injury by gradually reducing your heart rate and allowing your muscles to return to their resting state.

Reduces muscle soreness: When you exercise, your muscles produce lactic acid, which can cause soreness and fatigue. Cooling down and stretching can help flush out this lactic acid,

reducing muscle soreness and helping you
recover faster.

Improves flexibility: Stretching after exercise
can help improve your flexibility and range of
motion, making it easier for you to move and
perform daily activities.

Promotes relaxation: Cooling down and
stretching after exercise can help you relax and
reduce stress, which can have a positive impact
on your mental health.

Helps regulate blood flow: Cooling down after
exercise helps regulate blood flow, which can
help prevent dizziness and other symptoms that
can occur when you suddenly stop exercising.

Overall, cooling down and stretching after
exercise is an important part of any workout
routine. It helps you avoid injury, reduces
muscle soreness, improves flexibility, promotes
relaxation, and helps regulate blood flow.
Remember to always listen to your body and

stretch within your limits, and speak with your healthcare provider before starting any new exercise routine.

EXAMPLES OF EFFECTIVE COOL-DOWN EXERCISES FOR SENIORS

Cooling down is important for seniors after exercise as it helps them avoid injury, reduce muscle soreness, and regulate blood flow. Here are some examples of effective cool-down exercises for seniors:

Walking: Walking at a slower pace for 5-10 minutes after exercise can help seniors gradually reduce their heart rate and bring their body back to a resting state.

Gentle stretching: Stretching exercises, such as arm and leg swings, shoulder rolls, and neck stretches, can help seniors improve their flexibility and reduce muscle tension.

Yoga: Gentle yoga poses, such as the seated spinal twist, seated forward bend, and cat-cow stretch, can help seniors relax and stretch their muscles.

Tai Chi: This low-impact exercise involves slow, controlled movements that can help seniors improve their balance, coordination, and flexibility.

Deep breathing: Taking deep breaths and exhaling slowly can help seniors calm their mind and reduce stress.

Remember, it's important for seniors to cool down gradually and avoid sudden movements that could cause injury. It's also important to speak with a healthcare provider before starting any new exercise routine.

HOME WORKOUT ROUTINE CREATION
Creating a home workout routine can be an effective way to stay fit and healthy, especially if you don't have access to a gym or prefer to exercise in the comfort of your own home. Here

are some steps to help you create a home workout routine:

Assess your fitness level: Before starting any workout routine, it's important to assess your current fitness level. This can help you determine the intensity and duration of your workouts. You can consult with a personal trainer or use an online fitness test to evaluate your current fitness level.

Determine your goals: What do you want to achieve with your home workout routine? Are you trying to lose weight, build muscle, or improve your overall fitness level? Once you've identified your goals, you can create a workout plan that's tailored to your specific needs.

Choose your exercises: There are many different exercises you can do at home, including bodyweight exercises, yoga, Pilates, and cardio workouts. Choose exercises that align with your fitness goals and that you enjoy doing. It's important to include both strength training and cardio exercises in your routine for a well-rounded workout.

Plan your workout schedule: Decide how often you want to work out and schedule it into your daily routine. Consistency is key when it comes to seeing results, so try to stick to your workout schedule as much as possible.

Set realistic expectations: Don't expect to see results overnight. Building strength and improving fitness takes time and effort. Set realistic expectations and be patient with yourself.

Track your progress: Keep track of your workouts and your progress over time. This can help you stay motivated and see how far you've come.

Stay motivated: Finding the motivation to work out at home can be challenging, but there are many things you can do to stay motivated. Set short-term goals, reward yourself for reaching milestones, and find a workout buddy to keep you accountable.

By following these steps, you can create a home workout routine that fits your fitness goals and lifestyle. Remember to stay consistent and be patient, and you'll see the results you're looking for.

TIPS FOR CREATING A SAFE AND EFFECTIVE HOME WORKOUT ROUTINE FOR SENIORS OVER 60

Creating a safe and effective home workout routine for seniors over 60 requires some considerations to ensure that the exercise program is beneficial and safe for this age group. Here are some tips for creating a safe and effective home workout routine for seniors over 60:

Consult with a healthcare professional: Before starting any exercise program, it's important to consult with a healthcare professional to ensure that it's safe for you to exercise. This is especially important if you have any pre-existing medical conditions.

Start with low-impact exercises: Seniors over 60 should start with low-impact exercises such as walking, cycling, or swimming. These exercises are easier on the joints and can help improve cardiovascular health.

Focus on strength training: Strength training is important for seniors to maintain muscle mass and bone density. However, it's important to start with light weights and gradually increase the intensity as strength improves.

Incorporate balance exercises: Falls are a common cause of injury in seniors. Incorporating balance exercises, such as standing on one foot, can help improve balance and reduce the risk of falls.

Modify exercises as needed: Seniors may need to modify exercises to accommodate any physical limitations or injuries. For example, if you have knee problems, you may need to modify exercises that require bending the knees.

Use proper form: Using proper form is important to prevent injuries and ensure that exercises are effective. Consider working with a personal trainer or physical therapist to learn proper form.

Warm up and cool down: It's important to warm up before exercising and cool down after to prevent injury and reduce muscle soreness.

Stay hydrated: Seniors are more prone to dehydration, so it's important to drink plenty of water before, during, and after exercise.

By following these tips, seniors over 60 can create a safe and effective home workout routine that can improve their overall health and well-being. Remember to start slowly and gradually increase the intensity of the exercise program as strength and fitness improve.

HOW TO STAY MOTIVATED AND TRACK PROGRESS

Staying motivated and tracking progress is important to maintain a consistent workout routine and achieve your fitness goals. Here are some tips on how to stay motivated and track progress:

Set realistic goals: Setting realistic and achievable goals is important to stay motivated. Make sure your goals are specific, measurable, attainable, relevant, and time-bound (SMART).

Create a workout schedule: Scheduling your workouts in advance can help you stay on track and motivated. Treat your workouts like any other important appointment and stick to them as much as possible.

Find an accountability partner: Working out with a friend or hiring a personal trainer can help you stay accountable and motivated. Having someone to share your progress with and encourage you can help you stick to your workout routine.

Mix up your workouts: Doing the same workout routine can become boring and lead to loss of motivation. Mix up your workouts with different exercises, routines, or classes to keep things interesting and challenging.

Reward yourself: Setting up small rewards for achieving milestones or reaching your fitness goals can help you stay motivated. Rewards can be something as simple as treating yourself to a favorite meal or purchasing new workout gear.

Track your progress: Tracking progress can help you see how far you've come and motivate you to keep going. This can be done by keeping a workout log, taking progress photos, or using fitness tracking apps or wearable devices.

Celebrate your successes: Celebrating your successes, no matter how small, can help you stay motivated and positive. Recognize and celebrate your progress and achievements along the way.

Remember, staying motivated and tracking progress is a journey, not a destination. Celebrate your successes, learn from your setbacks, and keep going. With consistency and dedication, you can achieve your fitness goals.

MODIFICATIONS FOR DIFFERENT FITNESS LEVELS AND HEALTH CONDITIONS

When creating a home workout routine, it's important to consider modifications for different fitness levels and health conditions. Here are some general modifications that can be made to accommodate different fitness levels and health conditions:

Low-impact exercises: Low-impact exercises, such as walking, cycling, or swimming, can be easier on the joints and are suitable for seniors, individuals with joint problems, or those recovering from an injury.

Resistance bands or bodyweight exercises:
Resistance bands or bodyweight exercises can be
used as an alternative to weights for those who
are not ready to lift heavy weights or have
difficulty holding weights due to an injury or
joint pain.

Shorter workouts: For those who are just starting
or have a busy schedule, shorter workouts can be
effective. Breaking up workouts into shorter
sessions throughout the day can also be
beneficial.

Rest periods: Rest periods can be increased or
decreased depending on the individual's fitness
level. Beginners may need longer rest periods,
while those who are more advanced can shorten
the rest periods to increase the intensity of the
workout.

Modifications for health conditions: For those
with health conditions, modifications can be
made to exercises to accommodate their

condition. For example, those with back problems may need to modify exercises that require bending over or those with arthritis may need to modify exercises that put stress on the joints.

Personalized modifications: It's important to work with a healthcare professional or a certified personal trainer to create a personalized exercise program that takes into account individual health conditions and fitness levels.

Remember, it's important to listen to your body and modify exercises as needed to prevent injury and ensure that the workout is effective. By making modifications and adjustments, individuals of different fitness levels and health conditions can create a safe and effective home workout routine.

CONCLUSION

Regular exercise is important for everyone, but it becomes even more critical for seniors over 60.

As we age, our bodies naturally start to lose muscle mass, bone density, and flexibility. However, exercising regularly can help to slow down or even reverse these age-related changes, leading to improved health and quality of life.

Here are some of the benefits of regular exercise for seniors over 60

Improved cardiovascular health: Regular exercise can help to improve heart and lung function, reducing the risk of heart disease and stroke.

Increased muscle strength and balance: Exercise can help to build and maintain muscle mass, which is crucial for maintaining balance and preventing falls.

Enhanced flexibility: Regular stretching and flexibility exercises can help to improve joint mobility and reduce the risk of injury.

Better mood and mental health: Exercise releases endorphins, which can help to boost mood and reduce feelings of anxiety and depression.

Reduced risk of chronic diseases: Exercise has been shown to reduce the risk of chronic conditions such as diabetes, high blood pressure, and osteoporosis.

Improved sleep: Exercise can help to regulate the sleep-wake cycle and improve the quality of sleep.

It's important to note that seniors over 60 should always consult with a doctor before starting any new exercise program. A doctor can help to determine the best types of exercises based on a person's individual needs and health status. In general, seniors should aim for a mix of aerobic exercise (such as walking or cycling), strength training (such as lifting weights), and flexibility exercises (such as yoga or stretching) for optimal health benefits.

ENCOURAGEMENT TO START A SAFE AND EFFECTIVE HOME WORKOUT ROUTINE

Starting a safe and effective home workout routine can be an excellent way to improve your health and fitness. However, it can be challenging to get started, especially if you're new to exercising or don't know where to begin. Here are some tips to help you get started and stay motivated:

Start small: It's essential to start with a workout routine that is manageable and sustainable. Begin with short sessions of 10-15 minutes and gradually increase the length and intensity of your workouts.

Set achievable goals: Setting achievable goals can help you stay motivated and on track. Set realistic and achievable goals that are specific, measurable, and time-bound.

Find an exercise you enjoy: Exercise doesn't have to be boring or unenjoyable. Find a physical activity you enjoy, such as dancing, yoga, or cycling, and make it a part of your routine.

Make a plan: Plan out your workouts in advance, so you know exactly what exercises you'll be doing each day. This can help you stay on track and avoid procrastination.

Use resources: There are many resources available online to help you create a safe and effective workout routine, such as YouTube videos, fitness apps, and online fitness programs. Take advantage of these resources to help you achieve your fitness goals.

Stay motivated: Staying motivated is crucial to maintaining a consistent workout routine. Find a workout buddy or join an online fitness community to stay accountable and motivated.

Remember, starting a home workout routine is a great way to improve your health and fitness. However, it's important to start slowly, set achievable goals, and make a plan. Always consult with a doctor before starting any new exercise program, especially if you have any pre-existing medical conditions or concerns.